Halt Anxiety With Proven Techniques

Contents

Overview:

This book introduces techniques that help stop anxiety in its tracks every time you use them. An extensive body of research has reported each to be effective. Best of all, they are free to access anytime and anywhere.

Our body keeps us alive and well with two nervous systems that perform different roles: the sympathetic and the parasympathetic. We need them both to survive.

We need a fully operational sympathetic nervous system in situations where we must charge ahead and be in full control. Survival may be in question. When, for example you confront a bear when hiking in the forest or when managing 20 mentally ill employees, the sympathetic nervous system is your best friend and companion.

The end result, however, is emergence of over the top anxiety that is familiar to us all. Our parasympathetic nervous system is shut down for all practical purposes. The sympathetic system becomes so firmly in control and so domineering that the brakes required to disengage it have little if any effect. Fuel generated by the sympathetic system is adrenaline and cortisol and other "high intensity" hormones.

Anxiety is soothed by disengaging the full throttle of the sympathetic nervous system and re-engaging the dormant or less active parasympathetic nervous system.

The parasympathetic nervous system is needed for our body to generate dopamine and the other "rest and relax" and "chill out" hormones. The techniques I cover in this book settle down the sympathetic nervous system so that the parasympathetic nervous system can come "back on line."

When it comes down to getting relief from neurological symptoms the sympathetic nervous system is the "bully" of the relationship. Our parasympathetic is the "good" guy which is happy to always step aside and take a back seat when the sympathetic nervous system is in control. .

I think of the parasympathetic nervous system as the henpecked companion of the sympathetic. You will never succeed in calming down an overactive sympathetic nervous system by politely asking it to step aside.

OK. How in the world do you get the attention of the sympathetic nervous system to get out of the driver's seat take the back seat?

Halt Anxiety With Proven Techniques

We all are familiar with telling ourselves to calm down when we are nervous. You do not succeed by trying to force your frantic state of anxiety to step aside and "chill out." We are also all familiar with how trying to talk anxiety down can backfire and inflame an already anxious condition. It is all so frustrating.

But it does not have to be complicated to succeed. The following proven techniques are all simple to learn and simple to use. They instantly turn down the volume of an overactive sympathetic nervous system. Access them anytime and anywhere when anxiety is overwhelming and symptoms as driving you crazy. The connection between anxiety and symptoms is tight indeed.

There is one huge advantage to using these techniques to calm your anxiety. You get to celebrate the welcome benefit of quieting neurological symptoms.

Breathing

One powerful technique that calms down anxiety quickly is to breathe in a slightly different way. Why is breathing such an effective technique?

When we are afraid or when we are being traumatized, we freeze. We stop breathing altogether. This terminates horrible feelings that we cannot tolerate otherwise. When the horrible feelings are shut down, we are able to function in the face of terror. We can move through it. Stilling the breath makes it possible to survive in terrifying situations. Simply out - when we are scared we learn to stop breathing.

When we breathe, oxygen circulates through our body and the reverse happens. We are able to feel ourselves. We relax. We chill out. We feel safe.

Here is an explanation of a simple breathing technique that reduces anxiety.

> ***Take 3 breaths 3 times a day (at least). Make the breath when you inhale shorter than when you breathe out (the exhale). This results in an immediate relaxation reflex.***

Some breathing instructions to reduce anxiety will stipulate more specific instructions. For example, they recommend that you breathe in to the count of four (4) and breathe out to the count of six (6) - or breathe into the count of 4 and breath out to the count of 8.

It actually does not matter so much whether the count is 4 and 6 or something different. What matters is that the breath release is longer than the intake. The simple act of breathing deeply oxygenates our cells. This activates the relaxation reflex.

Visit the link below to hear audio clip explanations of this simple but highly effective anxiety reducing technique:

https://www.parkinsonsrecovery.com/reduce-anxiety-and-stress-with-breathing

Meditation

Meditation is a marvelous system for switching off the fight - flight sympathetic nervous system and switching on the rest and relaxation parasympathetic nervous system. It supports the natural production of those delicious hormones that help us fell yummy inside: dopamine, serotonin and melatonin. When our parasympathetic system is in charge, fewer medications and/or supplements are needed to suppress neurological symptoms. Meditation works wonders to accomplish this end.

There is a downside to relying on meditation as the only way to reduce anxiety. Effects are short lived.

An example will illustrate my point. Imagine that you have just spent 15 minutes in a deep altered state while meditating. Your body is relaxed. Your symptoms have been silenced. You are in that delicious zone of happiness.

Ten minutes later you receive an unexpected phone call from a family member who has just had a vehicle breakdown while driving on the interstate. They are stranded. They need your help.

What does this unexpected and distressing news do to you? Your body immediately shuts down the function of your parasympathetic nervous system and switches back on the sympathetic. As a result, adrenaline and cortisol flood the tissues of your body. These hormones are now in charge. And of course, you need to activate these hormones to address the emergency at hand.

Here is the rub: Not only are the "get up and go" hormones racing through the tissues of your body for a few hours but they linger in the body's tissues for as long as 48 hours. What happened to the chill out and relaxation hormones that your body manufactured while meditating? They are quickly exhausted. Their staying power is limited.

Everyone's life turns out to be full of daily stresses. Yes. Meditation is effective, but we cannot always stop our busy lives to meditate for 45 minutes. The breathing technique is helpful anytime and anywhere. You cannot meditate while changing a flat tire on the interstate. You can breathe.

I recommend you activate a combination of anxiety reduction techniques which include not only meditation, but breathing and the other techniques suggested in the following sections.

Want to learn more about how to meditate without making a big deal of it? Listen to the replay of my interview on September 24, 2009 with Norman Fischer by scrolling back pages here. All shows are in chronological order. http://www.blogtalkradio.com/parkinsons-recovery

Or, simply click on the link below:

Normal Fisher Discusses How to Meditate

Connection
A profound way to reduce anxiety is to connect deeply with another living being whether a person, animal or even plant. We usually connect with those we know well in

very familiar ways. When the connection shifts to a deeper level, anxiety is cut to the quick. Anxiety surfaces when we connect with another person who is not present.

For example, when encountering a family member or friend at the end of the day you may always ask them: "*What did you do today?*" The answer may typically be a cryptic summary of activities without mentioning a cruel backstabbing assault that occurred. In other words, the encounter is superficial.

Sometimes the connection is purely emotional.

With each new encounter – the question can be "how are you feeling today?" The answer may always be: "Fine". But, what you hear in such familiar interactions may be far removed from the truth. The person may be in a state of emotional turmoil.

The connection is superficial. Much of what is going on with a person is usually unexpressed. More often than not, a person will put on a smiley face – a mask of sorts – when they are actually depressed. What you see is not what is there.

Sometimes the connection is purely visual

What colors and clothes is a person wearing today? You form a quick judgment that their shoes are not polished. Why is the person wearing unpolished shoes? Don't they know better? First impressions keep us from having a more meaningful connection with other persons.

Perhaps this person was wearing the shoes their father once wore. The "truth" of the situation is that they simply wish to "walk" in their fathers shoes. Appearances often convey little truth.

Each of these "routine" examples of connection illustrates the superficial nature of how we often connect with others. But ….

Deeper Connections Calm Anxiety

Visit the following post for an audio explanation of what deeper connections entail:

https://www.parkinsonsrecovery.com/reduce-anxiety-and-stress-with-connection

Below is a detailed explanation of this proven technique:

Approach the next human being you encounter today differently.

How so?

The next person you see may be someone you see all the time.

- You likely have very familiar routines of interaction.

- This means that the two of you seldom become deeply connected with one another, much unlike when you meet a stranger for the first time (and especially so when the possibility of romance is involved).

Instead, form a deeper connection with them.

- Look them in the eyes.
- Reflect on what they are feeling.
- Speculate to yourself what they are not saying but thinking.
- Speculate to yourself what they are feeling but not expressing openly.
- Acknowledge your own feelings in the moment. Are you feeling weird or scattered or distant or happy or silly or what exactly?
- Why not confess how you are feeling?

This deeper connection need not involve dialogue.

- You are likely anticipating that the person you see next may respond with "*What is up with you*?" or "*Why are you acting so strangely*?"

If so, dialogue may not prove useful when it comes to having a more meaningful connection with friends and family. Form the connection at your end. They need not even be involved! Connection is all about reducing your anxiety. Deep connections with another do dissolve anxiety in its tracks

Deep connections do not have to involve another human being.

Connect with Pets or Wild Animals

You will be just as successful connecting with an animal – whether domestic or wild.

Connect with Plants

Plants are alive too just like humans and animals. Why not initiate a little chat with them?

Perhaps this sounds silly, but the most powerful and effective healer is nature.

- Hug a tree.
- Smell the flowers.
- Take a hike in the park.
- Swim in the ocean.

Nature always welcomes you. No invitations are required. Accept the perpetual invitation to treasure the natural world which is one step outside your home. In so doing, celebrate a quieting of anxiety.

Icy Cold Water

This next technique is a true winner when it comes to calming anxiety. I will first explain the magic of this technique by way of an analogy.

Computers sometimes fail us at the most critical times. We are trying to transmit an important and timely email, but our computer happens to be functioning at a snail's pace. It may be hours before the email send completes. What is wrong with your computer (or phone)? Anxiety begins to sizzle.

More than likely, a program on your computer is eating up processing capacity. Worse, it is a program that you did not even know was running, do not need and did not even start. How is this problem solved?

You must to terminate – switch off – the program that is eating up the processing capacity. Once you locate the program source and terminate it, your important email is transmitted immediately.

The icy water treatment offers a solution with a similar result. Its effect is immediate. It shuts down the program that is exhausting your energy. It shuts down your sympathetic nervous system which is "eating" up your energy and fueling your anxiety.

The icy water treatment quickly activates the parasympathetic nervous system. This in turn supports the body's ability to produce the rest and relaxation hormones of dopamine, serotonin and melatonin naturally which of course is why symptoms are calmed along with anxiety.

After all, if you want to turn someone off, don't you give them the Icy Water Treatment? It works for me every time.

Here is how to set it up so that it is available when needed. For an audio explanation visit the following:

https://www.parkinsonsrecovery.com/step-five-reduce-anxiety-using-icy-cold-water-treatment

1. Find a bowl large enough for your hands to fit inside:

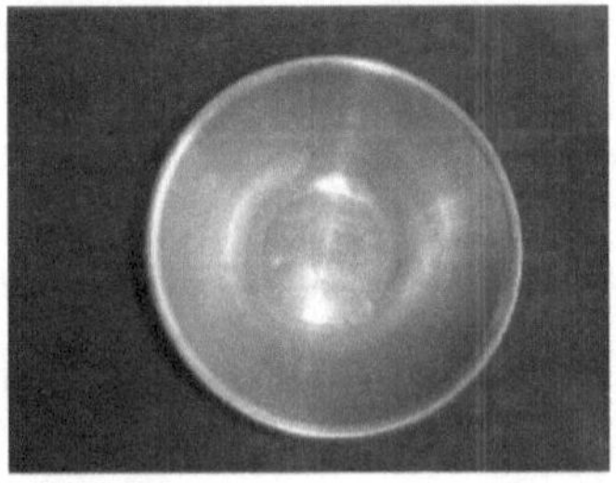

2. Grab an Ice Cube Tray or collect ice

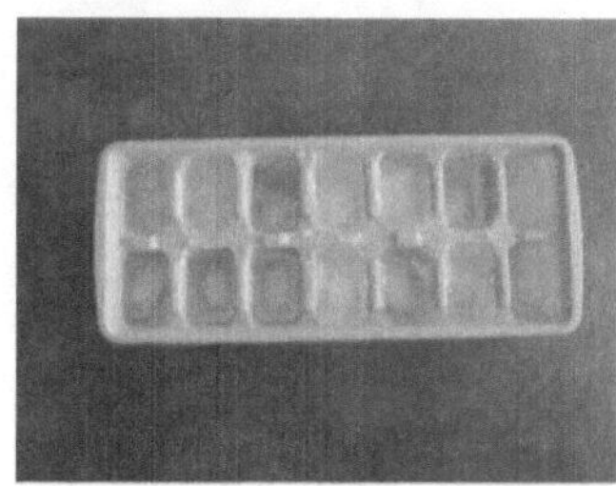

3. Fill the bowl half way up with water. .

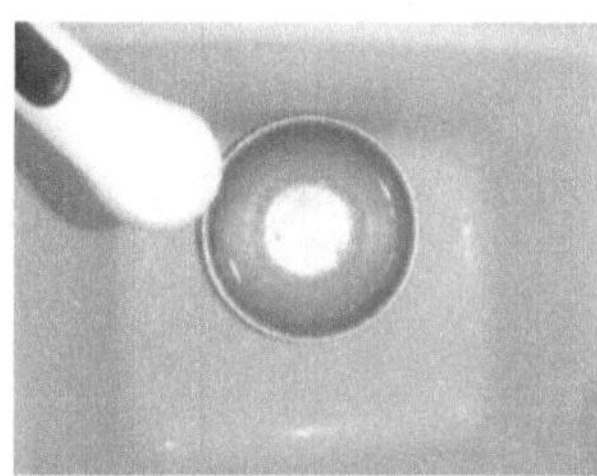

4. Put some ice cubes in the water. .

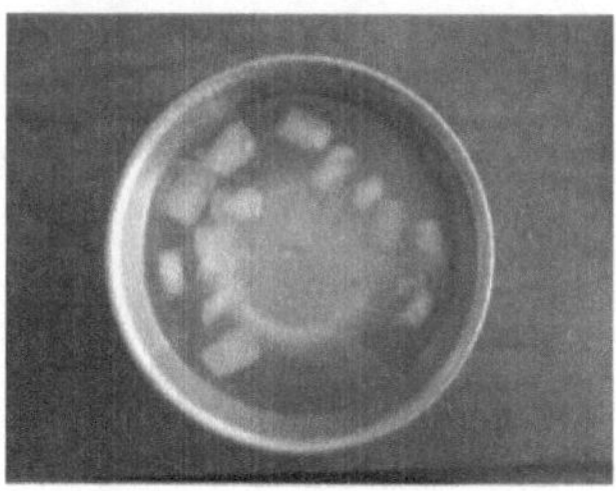

5. When feeling anxious, immerse your two hands into the icy cold water for 10-15 seconds (or longer if you can tolerate it

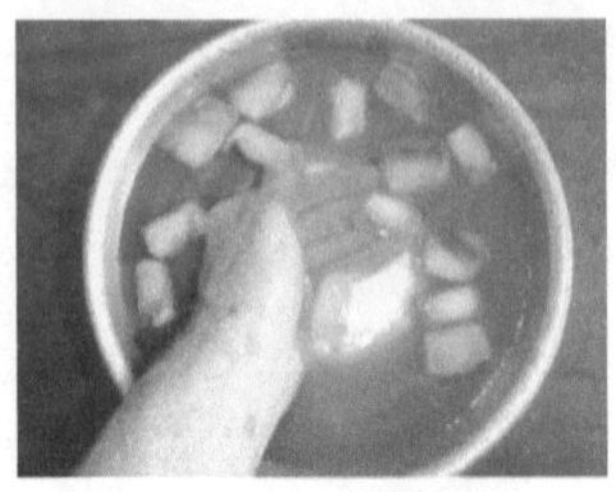

It is as easy as that!

Keep the bowl of cold water handy and readily available at home when you need it. Why not just put the bowl of icy cold water in the fridge? You can use this as many times a day as needed.

What do you do when your bowl of icy cold water is not accessible? When you leave home, bring a small wash rag with you. Why? When you need to calm down anxiety that begins to wreak havoc on your sanity, wet the wash rag in cold water (available in any bathroom) and wipe your face with it. That will reduce your anxiety level too.

Halt Anxiety With Proven Techniques

New Year Day Dip in the Icy Cold Water

I suspect you have observed or heard about people who every New Year day take a quick dip in their chilly town lake or river to celebrate the coming of the new year . The truth of this somewhat strange behavior is that it sets them in motion to release the anxieties of the past year so that the events of the New Year can be embraced and celebrated. They intentionally shut down their sympathetic nervous system to make way for a new beginning.   There really is a sound rational to this seemingly crazy ritual.

Cold Strengthens the Immune System

Here is another good reason to take the cold water treatment seriously. Wim Hof is known as the 'Iceman.' He routinely subjects his body to bouts of extremely cold temperatures which stimulate his immune and cardiovascular system.

It is well known that too much cortisol (generated by an overactive sympathetic nervous system) weakens our immune system. The Icy Water Treatment does the reverse. The production is cortisol is shut down because the sympathetic nervous system is turned off (temporality).

Wim argues that the cold is your friend. Regular exposure to the cold strengthens the immune system. Most of us avoid exposure to the cold and treasure the comforts of home. When we become cold we immediately crank up the heating system or put on sweaters. Capillaries and veins are not able to function as originally intended. Wim argues that when the cold is embraced, magic begins to happen. It opens up the tiny capillaries which are better able to transport nutrients to the cells and remove waste products from them.

Consider adding to your daily ritual an icy cold water rinse in your shower. This will shock your immune system into becoming stronger and more resilient. This will also make it easier for your body to fend off noxious infections and viruses. Or hey – why not take a dip in the cold water every New Year's?

Grounding

The next techniques to be introduced and explained accomplish the same thing but in different ways. They both "ground" you. What in the world am I talking about here?

When anxious, energy is spewing out of control. We all know the feeling. Everything feels out of sorts and scattered. We are not ourselves. No task however small is easy to accomplish. We encounter problems no matter where we turn.

When we are anxious, feeling "out of sorts" and "outside of our body", our energy is sparking around our head in every which direction and circling around the top of our body - not our legs and feet.

Have you ever come across an electrical wire that was snapped in a storm and is flapping about in the air? You can see electrical sparks when this happens. The loose wire is not grounded.

This is precisely what the energy looks like to healers who see sparks of energy spewing out of your head in all directions. It swirls about like a hurricane around when you are anxious.

- Why do people who are continuously anxious feel off balance so often?
- Why do some have perplexing mobility challenges?
- Worse – why do some fall frequently?

The Answer:

They are energetically top heavy. Simply put – most of their energy is spinning haphazardly around the top of their body. Little energy is present at the bottom of their body. When we (or a boat floating in the water) is top heavy it is more prone to falls and tipping over.

The solution to these problems is grounding.

To ground a loose wire you have to connect the wire to a metal post in the ground or insulate it. And when you are anxious, that is precisely what you need to do. Shift the chaotic energy (which is full of sparks swirling around your head) down to your feet. This feat requires grounding.

The following DVD presents a fascinating presentation that illustrates the value of grounding in a small community in Alaska.

https://grounded.com/the-grounded-movie/

The two following simple techniques shift upper body energy fueling the anxiety to the lower body. This shift provides the grounding that is needed. It takes little time to take effect.

This by the way is why you always feel so much better when you hug a tree. Trees are grounded because their roots are permanently connected to the earth. Hugging trees can always help us become better grounded.

Butt Squeeze

When you are anxious squeeze your butt muscles. You can do this anywhere - any time - without anyone even knowing you are doing it. Keep squeezing until you feel a noticeable relief from feeling anxious.

That is it folks. Do not think about it. Just do it. This simple technique really is extracted from the research which describes it in a rather convoluted manner. We modified the technique to make it simple to use without having to remember which muscles need to be squeezed.

Feet Focus

You can also ground by looking down at your feet. Now that is simple, eh? Better yet, you can rock and swish each foot to insure that the grounding is sustained for a longer period. It does not take much for anyone to become ungrounded which can happen instantly.

There are three movements for each foot. Do each of the movements eight times each.

1. With your toes firmly anchored on the ground, rotate your heel 8 times clockwise and 8 times counterclockwise.

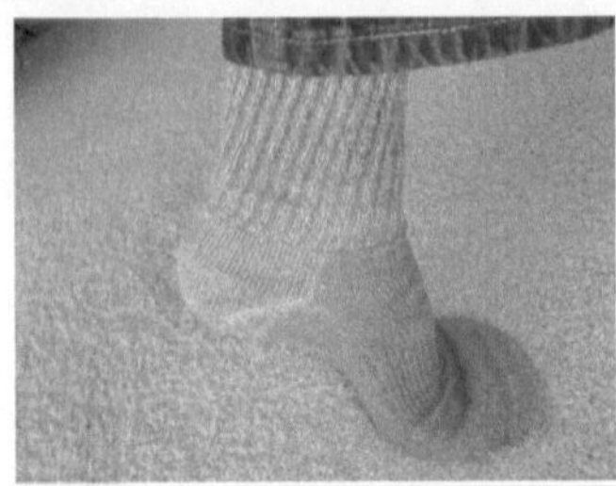

Now do the same using the other foot.

2. Rock your foot back and forth - first with your toes on the ground and heel in the air, then with your heel on the ground and toes in the air. Do this 8 times on each foot.

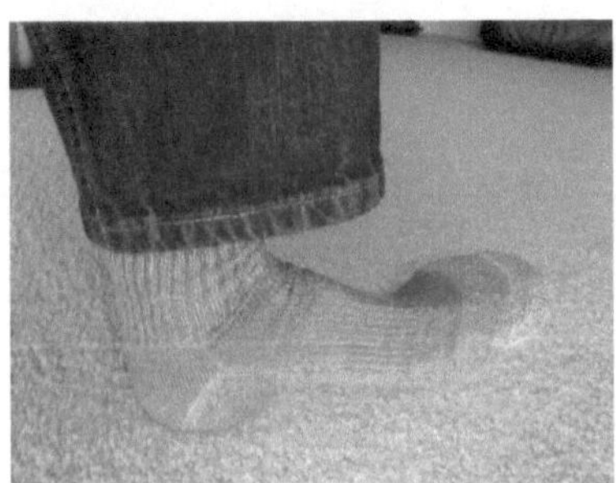

3. Swish each foot 8 times back and forth.

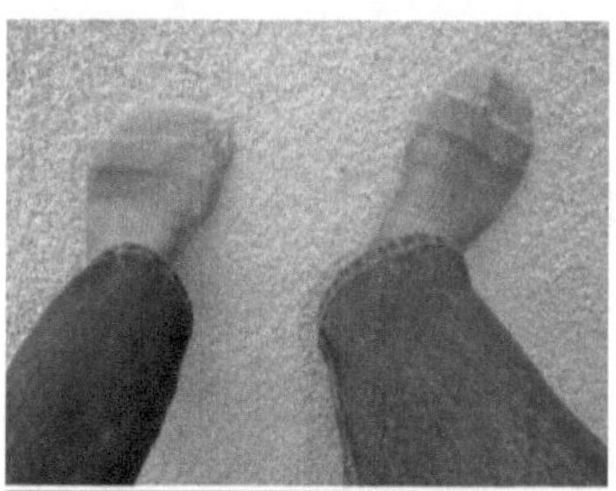

Slow Down

Give yourself the gift of taking extra time to accomplish each and every task throughout each day. When stressed and anxious, our minds and bodies are churning on overdrive. We can become so frantic that we sometimes have to admit to ourselves we are "out of control."

- Instead of moving mindfully, we are trying to "race" from one destination to another.

- It feels that there is not enough time and that there has never been enough time…too much to do … too little time to do it all.

- We make plans of what to accomplish, but few items on our list are ever completed by the end of the day.

Familiar solutions are…

1. Move faster
2. Do everything more quickly

They will inevitably inflame symptoms because anxiety becomes so problematic.

My solution to the problems that rushing creates for us is simple:

Slow Everything In Your Life Down

Always take extra time to accomplish each and every task. For example, having guests over for dinner Friday night? Perhaps you could get everything ready for the dinner Friday night beginning at 2:00 in the afternoon Friday when you were younger. But anxiety has become problematic and symptoms themselves always slow you down. Start planning for your Friday night party three days in advance (or longer).

- No racing or rushing to get ready for the party.
- No worries that there is not enough time to prepare food for the dinner or clean the house.

Allot extra time to prepare slowly and mindfully even it means you start getting ready for the party a week before.

This rule applies to every task.

Have an appointment with a doctor?

> Triple the time you think it will take to get there. Start early. Enjoy the commute. It is stressful enough to see a doctor in the first place. Why accelerate your anxiety when you discover you are going to be late for your appointment?

Stop Multi-Tasking

This suggestion will admittedly be more difficult for women than men. Women are so much better at multi-tasking than men.

This means: Do not fix a meal and listen to the radio (or watch television) at the same time. Focus entirely on fixing the meal. Or, focus exclusively on listening to the radio or watching TV.

- When eating a meal – only eat. Do not also look at your smart phone.
- When talking with a friend on the phone – do not also fold the laundry or munch on an apple.

Commit to doing one and only one task at a time. Why? You get anxiety under better control and celebrate a quieting of symptoms.

You may be thinking – but I will really not have enough time now if I cannot multi-task. It has always worked for me in the past. Right - but not now if anxiety is an issue.

Might I now suggest that you will have more time because stress and anxiety will no longer fuel your symptoms.

Isn't getting relief from symptoms worth changing a few lifelong habits that no longer serve your best and highest good?

Perhaps you have tried in the past to minimize or eliminate multi-tasking with little success. For you, It is irritating to attend to one and only one task like listening to one of Robert's radio show interviews and doing nothing else. Why not surf the internet too while listening? So much more can be accomplished, right?

I say wrong. The restless energy you are experiencing lies at the root cause of neurological symptoms. I suggest that if you resist my suggestion to minimize multi-tasking because it is too "boring," meditate on why you are feeling bored and restless.

Think of the challenge as similar to hugging a child who is so worked up they cannot go to sleep at night. Your nervous system can also not turn off. When you connect deeply with that place deep inside of where restlessness resides, you will at long last connect with the root cause of your symptoms.

Connection, as you now know, is what reduces anxiety. In this case, you are connecting with yourself rather than another person.

Resist the temptation to multitask. Acknowledge the feeling of restlessness.

- Hug yourself.
- Hold yourself.
- Observe your body relax.

Celebrate how anxiety dissolves and symptoms become less problematic.

Just Say No

A persistent trigger of anxiety is doing something that we resent.

- *We get irritated.*
- *We become angry*
- *We are rattled with resentment.*

Now, most of us do not usually let our feelings be known but this does not silence their impact. They fuel anxiety and sustain symptoms. How can we avoid such unpleasant thoughts and feelings?

Just Say No. Do not do it!

You find yourself doing something – not because it gives you joy and nourishment – but because it is expected. For example, perhaps it has always been your "job" to make the bed. Your spouse expects it. Your spouse likes a tidy bed. More and more however, you resent having to make up the bed every day. Why not –

Just say no! I am not doing this anymore.

You observe yourself doing something – not because it gives you joy and nourishment – but because you have always done it. For example, perhaps you have always driven to the bank every month to deposit your check. It is a task you have come to dislike because the traffic has become unmanageable. Why not arrange an alternative solution like getting your funds transferred automatically. In other words, why not –

Just say no. I am not doing this anymore.

STARS

This powerful technique does not suggest that you "hang out" with the stars to reduce anxiety. That would surely un-ground you!

STARS letters stand for:::

> **See**
>
> **Touch**
>
> **Auditory**
>
> **Remember**
>
> **Smell**

STARS is a simple way to recall the benefits of a successful mindfulness practice. Research is unequivocal: Mindfulness offers a sure fire ability to cut anxiety to the quick.

The guiding theme of mindfulness is to shut down the hamster wheel of worrisome thoughts that cause high anxiety by bringing yourself totally and completely into the present moment.

This is a place where you have no regrets about the past. It can never be changed. And, this is a place where you have no worries and frets about the future. After all, how often are your projections about what will happen in the future realized?

The idea, simply put, is to focus 100% of your immediate attention on "taking in" totally and completely every aspect of your surroundings (even if you are in very familiar surroundings like your living room).

- What objects do you notice? Are they thick, thin, sharp dull and so on …, etc?

- What is your body touching in the moment (feet on the ground, hands on a table, etc.?) How does the touch feel (cold, hot, clammy, smooth, etc.)?

- What sounds do you hear (birds chirping, people talking, machines vibrating, etc.)?

- When you move from one space to another, what do you remember about the previous space? What were the colors of the clothes people were wearing? What was on the walls of the room you were just in?
- What were the sounds?
- What are the smells in the space?

In other words, activate all of the senses

See it

Touch it

Hear~~hear~~ it

(Auditory~~auditory~~)

Remember it

Smell it

Gift of Waiting

Do you get irritated and even angry when you have to wait a long time? Consider a different emotional response to when you have to wait for service.

How so?

This is the perfect opportunity to become mindful in the moment. If you have to wait in a long line …

What are the expressions on the faces of others who are waiting along with you?

- *Are they angry?*
- *Mad?*
- *Irritated?*
- *What color are their shoes … their clothes?*
- *What are they holding in their hands?*
- *What noises do you hear while you are waiting?*
- *What are the smells?*
- *What does the ceiling look like?*

OK. I could ask hundreds of questions to ponder here. You get the point.

When you focus on supporting and strengthening an ongoing mindfulness practice (which means in effect you are mindful throughout the day) you will get the welcome benefit of celebrating a quieting of symptoms.

Benefits are unbeatable:

No side effects

No expense involved

You are in control

Your senses are heightened

Your overall joy of living is enhanced

Symptoms are less problematic

Mindfulness Series

Visit the link below for information about a series of mindfulness challenges specially designed for persons with neurological challenges:

https://www.parkinsonsrecovery.com/mindfulness

Robert Rodgers PhD

Olympia Washington

Road to Recovery from Parkinsons Disease

https://www.parkinsonsdisease.me